MEDICAL ETHICS POCKET GUIDE

DR. MOHAMED ELGENDY
LMCC, CCFP
CANADA

DISCLAIMER

This pocket guide was developed with the assistance of advanced AI tools to streamline content generation. Every chapter has been thoroughly reviewed, edited, and authenticated by Dr. Mohamed Elgendy, LMCC, CCFP (Canada), ensuring accuracy, credibility, and clinical authenticity. The result is a modern, innovative reference that blends the efficiency of AI with the rigor of professional medical expertise

This booklet is intended for educational purposes only and should not be used as a substitute for professional legal, ethical, or clinical advice. Although based on Canadian guidelines and ethical principles, individual circumstances, jurisdictional laws, and institutional policies may vary. Clinicians are advised to consult appropriate regulatory bodies, ethics committees, or legal counsel when dealing with complex or high-risk cases.

The author and publisher accept no liability for the consequences of decisions made based on this content.

ABOUT THE AUTHOR

Dr. Mohamed Elgendy is a licensed Canadian physician with the Licentiate of the Medical Council of Canada (LMCC) and Certification in Family Medicine (CCFP) from the College of Family Physicians of Canada. He has several years of hands-on experience as both a rural emergency physician and a family doctor, currently practicing in Saskatchewan, Canada. With a deep commitment to improving healthcare delivery in underserved communities, Dr. Elgendy focuses on practical, evidence-based medicine tailored to the realities of rural practice. His work bridges the gap between academic medicine and frontline care, offering accessible resources to help clinicians make confident, life-saving decisions in resource-limited settings

With this *Medical Ethics Pocket Guide,* Dr. Elgendy aims to provide medical learners and clinicians with a concise, practical resource that bridges the gap between theory and the daily ethical challenges faced in patient care. His work reflects a passion for empowering healthcare providers to deliver safe, ethical, and patient-centered care across diverse practice environments

DEDICATION

This book is dedicated to the patients in rural and remote communities, whose dignity, values, and trust guide every decision we make; to the healthcare providers who navigate complex ethical challenges with integrity, compassion, and respect, often in resource-limited settings; and to my family, whose unwavering support and understanding make this work possible.

— Dr. Mohamed Elgendy

TABLE OF CONTENTS

CHAPTER 1
Access to Care and Health Equity

Definition:

Access to care refers to the ability of individuals to obtain timely and appropriate healthcare services. Health equity ensures that care is distributed fairly, recognizing and addressing barriers linked to social determinants of health, such as income, geography, race, or disability. Promoting health equity is a core ethical obligation for healthcare providers and systems.

Case Scenario (Ethical Dilemma):

Ms. A, a 47-year-old woman with unstable housing and no primary care provider, presents repeatedly to the emergency department for uncontrolled diabetes. Some staff express frustration, referring to her as a 'frequent flyer.' She misses specialist appointments due to transportation issues. Dr. Malik wonders how to address her medical needs without reinforcing stigma or system overuse.

Question:

How can Dr. Malik uphold ethical obligations related to access and equity in caring for Ms. A?

Answer:

Dr. Malik should provide respectful, nonjudgmental care while advocating for system-level supports that improve equitable access (e.g., social work, community outreach, housing referrals).

Explanation:

Ethical care involves recognizing the impact of structural and social barriers on health. Providers must avoid stigmatizing language and advocate for vulnerable patients. Interventions that link patients with wraparound supports and address determinants of health are key to promoting equity. Clinicians also have a role in calling for broader health system reforms.

References:

- Canadian Medical Association (CMA): Health Equity and Access Framework
- World Health Organization: Social Determinants of Health
- Canadian Medical Protective Association (CMPA): Addressing Barriers to Care
- Health Quality Ontario: Equity in Healthcare Access

CHAPTER 2
Advance Directives and Goals of Care

Definition:

Advance directives are written or verbal instructions that communicate a patient's preferences for medical care in the event they become incapable of making decisions. Goals of care discussions involve identifying what matters most to the patient and aligning medical interventions with their values, especially near end-of-life.

Case Scenario (Ethical Dilemma):

Mr. Zhang, an 89-year-old man with metastatic pancreatic cancer, is brought to the emergency department in septic shock. He is intubated and admitted to the ICU. His daughter brings a written advance directive signed last year stating he does not wish to be intubated or resuscitated. The ICU team was unaware of this document at the time of intubation. Now stabilized, he remains sedated and cannot be extubated immediately. The family is upset and demands immediate withdrawal of life support.

Question:

How should the ICU team proceed in light of Mr. Zhang's advance directive and current condition?

Answer:

The team should urgently review and honor Mr. Zhang's advance directive and engage the family in shared decision-making. Immediate withdrawal may not be medically safe, but the goals of care should shift toward comfort-oriented measures.

Explanation:

Advance directives are ethically and legally binding if they are valid and applicable. Although the team initially acted without knowledge of the directive, they must now realign care with the patient's previously expressed wishes. The timing and manner of withdrawal should balance clinical safety and respect for autonomy. Goals-of-care discussions with the family help clarify the plan moving forward, emphasizing palliative approaches aligned with the patient's values.

References:

- Canadian Medical Association (CMA) Code of Ethics and Professionalism
- Canadian Hospice Palliative Care Association: Advance Care Planning Guide
- College of Physicians and Surgeons of Ontario (CPSO): Planning for and Providing Quality End-of-Life Care
- CMPA: Advance Care Planning and Goals of Care

CHAPTER 3
Allocation of Scarce Resources (e.g., ICU beds, transplant organs)

Definition:

The allocation of scarce medical resources involves making difficult decisions about which patients receive limited treatments such as ICU beds or organ transplants. Ethical principles guiding allocation include fairness, equity, medical utility, transparency, and respect for persons.

Case Scenario (Ethical Dilemma):

During a COVID-19 surge, only one ICU bed remains available. Two patients require admission: a 45-year-old with a high chance of recovery and a 78-year-old with multiple comorbidities but who has been a community leader and requests full treatment. The ICU triage team must decide who gets the bed. The older patient's family argues that social contributions should influence the decision.

Question:

What ethical principles should guide the triage team's decision, and is it appropriate to consider social worth in this context?

Answer:

Allocation should prioritize medical need and likelihood of benefit. Social worth should not be a criterion for resource allocation.

Explanation:

Ethical resource allocation relies on principles such as maximizing benefit (e.g., survival), treating people equally, and prioritizing the worst off when feasible. Using social value can lead to discrimination and undermine fairness. Transparent, evidence-based triage protocols help avoid bias and maintain public trust, especially in crises.

References:

- Canadian Medical Association (CMA) Framework on Ethical Allocation of Resources
- Ontario COVID-19 Bioethics Table: Triage Protocol for ICU Admission
- Canadian Medical Protective Association (CMPA): Ethics of Resource Scarcity
- Beauchamp TL, Childress JF. Principles of Biomedical Ethics. 8th ed. Oxford University Press; 2019.

CHAPTER 4
Artificial Intelligence and Decision Support in Medicine – Ethical Considerations

Definition

Artificial Intelligence (AI) in medicine refers to the use of algorithms, machine learning models, and automated decision-support systems to assist clinicians in diagnosis, treatment planning, and patient monitoring. Ethical considerations include transparency, accountability, bias in algorithms, patient consent for AI use, and the physician's duty to maintain clinical judgment despite technological recommendations.

Case Scenario (Ethical Dilemma)

A 58-year-old man presents with chest discomfort. The rural emergency department recently implemented an AI-driven ECG interpretation tool that flags potential acute myocardial infarction cases. The AI system reports 'likely STEMI,' but the physician reviewing the ECG disagrees based on ST segment morphology and clinical context. The patient asks, 'Shouldn't we just follow what the computer says? It must be right.' The physician now faces the challenge of explaining the decision while ensuring patient safety and maintaining trust.

Question

What ethical obligations does the physician have when AI recommendations conflict with clinical judgment?

Answer

The physician should integrate AI-generated recommendations into the decision-making process but must retain ultimate responsibility for patient care, applying independent clinical judgment. AI should be treated as a support tool, not a replacement for human expertise.

Explanation

- Patient Safety First: Physicians must prioritize patient welfare over adherence to automated suggestions, especially if clinical evidence suggests a different course of action.
- Transparency: Clearly communicate to the patient that AI is a decision-support tool, not an infallible authority.
- Informed Consent: Patients should be aware if AI technology is being used in their care and understand its limitations.
- Bias and Data Quality: AI systems are only as good as the data they are trained on; bias or outdated information can lead to errors.
- Accountability: Legal and ethical responsibility for decisions remains with the clinician, even if AI tools are used.
- Continuous Learning: Clinicians should remain up-to-date on AI capabilities, limitations, and regulatory standards.

CHAPTER 5
Breaking Bad News

Definition:

Breaking bad news is the process of delivering information that may cause a patient emotional distress, such as the diagnosis of a serious illness or a poor prognosis. It requires sensitivity, empathy, clear communication, and respect for the patient's emotional and informational needs.

Case Scenario (Ethical Dilemma):

Dr. Ahmed is caring for Mrs. Li, a 68-year-old woman recently diagnosed with metastatic lung cancer. Her son approaches Dr. Ahmed before the disclosure and asks him not to tell his mother the full diagnosis, fearing it will cause her emotional harm. Mrs. Li, however, has previously expressed a desire to know the full truth about her health. Dr. Ahmed is unsure how to proceed.

Question:

Should Dr. Ahmed honor the son's request or disclose the full diagnosis to Mrs. Li?

Answer:

Dr. Ahmed should respect Mrs. Li's prior expressed wishes and disclose the diagnosis in a compassionate and clear manner.

Explanation:

Patients have the right to know about their health, especially if they have previously stated a desire to be informed. While family concerns may be valid, they do not override the principle of patient autonomy. Dr. Ahmed should prepare a quiet, private setting, assess Mrs. Li's readiness to receive information, and use a structured approach (e.g., SPIKES protocol) to deliver the news with empathy and support.

References:

- SPIKES Protocol for Breaking Bad News (Baile et al., 2000)
- Canadian Medical Protective Association (CMPA): Communicating Difficult News
- Canadian Medical Association (CMA) Code of Ethics and Professionalism
- College of Physicians and Surgeons of Ontario (CPSO): Effective Physician-Patient Communication

CHAPTER 6
Capacity and Decision-Making

Definition:

Capacity refers to a patient's ability to understand and appreciate the nature and consequences of a health-related decision. It is task-specific and can vary over time. Assessing capacity is essential in determining whether a patient can give informed consent or refuse treatment.

Case Scenario (Ethical Dilemma):

Ms. Robinson, an 83-year-old woman with moderate dementia, is admitted to the hospital with a hip fracture. She needs urgent surgery. She expresses confusion about the procedure but clearly says she doesn't want an operation. Her son insists she undergo surgery and says she is 'not in her right mind' to refuse. The orthopedic team is unsure whether her refusal should be respected or overridden.

Question:

How should the healthcare team assess and proceed regarding Ms. Robinson's capacity to refuse surgery?

Answer:

The team must perform a formal assessment of Ms. Robinson's decision-making capacity. If she is deemed capable, her decision to refuse surgery must be respected.

Explanation:

Capacity is not determined by diagnosis (e.g., dementia) alone, but by evaluating whether the patient understands relevant information, can appreciate the consequences of their choice, and can communicate a decision. If Ms. Robinson meets these criteria, she has the right to refuse surgery, even if the decision carries risk. If she lacks capacity, a substitute decision-maker (e.g., her son) may consent on her behalf in accordance with legal and ethical standards.

References:

- College of Physicians and Surgeons of Ontario (CPSO): Policy on Consent and Capacity
- Canadian Medical Protective Association (CMPA): Determining Capacity to Consent
- Health Care Consent Act (Ontario), 1996
- Canadian Medical Association (CMA) Code of Ethics and Professionalism

CHAPTER 7
Confidentiality and Privacy

Definition:

Confidentiality refers to the ethical and legal duty of healthcare professionals to protect personal health information entrusted to them. Privacy relates to the patient's right to control access to their personal and medical information. Both are essential to maintaining trust in the healthcare relationship.

Case Scenario (Ethical Dilemma):

Dr. Singh is treating a 19-year-old university student, Sarah, for depression. Her mother calls the clinic asking for updates on Sarah's treatment, expressing concern over recent changes in her daughter's mood. Sarah has not given permission to share any details with her family. Dr. Singh is unsure whether to respect Sarah's confidentiality or share information with her worried mother.

Question:

Is Dr. Singh permitted to share information with Sarah's mother without her explicit consent?

Answer:

No. Dr. Singh is ethically and legally obligated to maintain Sarah's confidentiality unless there is imminent risk of harm or Sarah consents to disclosure.

Explanation:

Patients over the age of majority who are capable of making their own medical decisions are entitled to full confidentiality, regardless of parental concern. Disclosure without consent is only permissible if there is a serious and imminent threat to the patient or others. Dr.

Singh should encourage Sarah to involve her family if appropriate but must prioritize her autonomy and privacy.

References:

- Personal Health Information Protection Act (PHIPA), Ontario
- Canadian Medical Protective Association (CMPA): Confidentiality and Privacy
- College of Physicians and Surgeons of Ontario (CPSO): Protecting Personal Health Information
- Canadian Medical Association (CMA) Code of Ethics and Professionalism

CHAPTER 8
Conflict of Interest

Definition:

A conflict of interest in healthcare arises when a physician's personal, financial, or professional interests could compromise—or appear to compromise—their judgment, integrity, or responsibility to act in the best interests of their patients.

Case Scenario (Ethical Dilemma):

Dr. Santos is participating in a clinical trial funded by a pharmaceutical company for a new diabetes medication. She receives honoraria for speaking about the drug at conferences. A newly diagnosed patient asks whether to start this new drug or a well-established alternative. Dr. Santos believes the new drug has promise, but she also knows her professional relationship with the sponsor could raise concerns.

Question:

How should Dr. Santos manage this situation to uphold ethical standards and protect patient trust?

Answer:

Dr. Santos must disclose the potential conflict of interest to the patient and provide unbiased, evidence-based information about all treatment options.

Explanation:

Physicians must prioritize the patient's best interests and maintain transparency when a potential or perceived conflict of interest exists. Disclosure allows patients to make informed decisions and helps preserve trust. Physicians should avoid promoting treatments where their impartiality could be questioned and should rely on clinical evidence and guidelines.

References:

- Canadian Medical Association (CMA) Code of Ethics and Professionalism
- Canadian Medical Protective Association (CMPA): Conflict of Interest Advice
- College of Physicians and Surgeons of Ontario (CPSO): Conflict of Interest Policy
- World Medical Association: Declaration of Geneva and Guidelines on Physician-Industry Relationships

CHAPTER 9
Cultural Sensitivity and Respect for Indigenous Health Practices

Definition:

Cultural sensitivity in healthcare involves recognizing, respecting, and responding to the unique values, beliefs, and practices of diverse populations. In the context of Indigenous health, it includes understanding the impact of colonialism, honoring traditional healing practices, and fostering culturally safe care that supports reconciliation and autonomy.

Case Scenario (Ethical Dilemma):

A Cree elder, Mr. W., is hospitalized with advanced heart failure. He requests to leave the hospital temporarily to participate in a traditional sweat lodge ceremony, which he believes is essential for his healing. The cardiologist is concerned about his unstable condition and discourages the ceremony, advising against discharge. Mr. W. insists this ceremony aligns with his spiritual needs and cultural identity.

Question:

How should the healthcare team address Mr. W.'s request while balancing medical risk and cultural respect?

Answer:

The healthcare team should engage in shared decision-making, exploring how to support Mr. W.'s cultural and spiritual needs while minimizing clinical risk. Refusal without dialogue undermines culturally safe care.

Explanation:

Respecting Indigenous health practices requires cultural humility and a trauma-informed approach. Healthcare providers must avoid paternalism and seek collaborative solutions, such as arranging safe participation in ceremony or involving cultural liaisons or Indigenous Elders. Providing culturally respectful care promotes trust and supports reconciliation in the healthcare system.

References:

- Truth and Reconciliation Commission of Canada: Calls to Action (Health)
- Indigenous Services Canada: Cultural Safety and Humility Guidelines
- Canadian Medical Association (CMA) Policy on Indigenous Health
- National Collaborating Centre for Indigenous Health (NCCIH): Culturally Safe Care Resources

CHAPTER 10
Do Not Resuscitate (DNR) Orders

Definition:

A Do Not Resuscitate (DNR) order is a medical directive indicating that cardiopulmonary resuscitation (CPR) should not be attempted if a patient experiences cardiac or respiratory arrest. DNR orders are based on the patient's preferences, prognosis, and overall goals of care, and must be clearly documented and communicated.

Case Scenario (Ethical Dilemma):

Mr. Green, a 74-year-old man with advanced metastatic cancer, has a documented DNR order in his hospital chart. During morning rounds, he suddenly collapses in his hospital room. A newly rotated medical resident, unaware of the DNR status, begins full CPR. The code team arrives and revives Mr. Green. The family is distraught and questions how this happened.

Question:

Was initiating CPR in this situation ethically and procedurally appropriate? What should be done to prevent such incidents?

Answer:

No, CPR should not have been initiated given the valid DNR order. This represents a breakdown in communication and handover processes.

Explanation:

DNR orders must be clearly documented, accessible, and effectively communicated to all members of the healthcare team. Failure to respect a DNR order can cause patient and family distress and violates the patient's autonomy. To prevent such events, teams must improve handover protocols, post visible DNR indicators where appropriate, and ensure all clinicians review resuscitation status during patient care transitions.

References:

- Canadian Medical Protective Association (CMPA): DNR Orders and Communication
- College of Physicians and Surgeons of Ontario (CPSO): Planning for and Providing Quality End-of-Life Care
- Canadian Medical Association (CMA) Code of Ethics and Professionalism
- National DNR Guidelines – Canadian Critical Care Society (CCCS)

CHAPTER 11
Duty to Treat vs. Physician Safety During Infectious Disease Outbreaks

Definition:

The ethical conflict between a physician's duty to provide care to patients and the need to protect their own health and safety during infectious disease outbreaks. This issue often arises during pandemics or localized epidemics where the risk of transmission to healthcare providers is significant.

Case Scenario (Ethical Dilemma):

Dr. L is working in a community hospital during an outbreak of a highly contagious respiratory virus. The hospital is facing a shortage of personal protective equipment (PPE). A critically ill patient requires immediate intubation, a procedure known to generate infectious aerosols. Without full PPE, Dr. L faces a high risk of infection but delaying the procedure could lead to the patient's death.

Question:

Should Dr. L proceed with the intubation despite the lack of adequate PPE, or should they wait until proper protection is available, knowing it could cost the patient's life?

Answer:

Ethically, the physician must balance their professional duty to treat with the obligation to maintain their own health and avoid becoming a source of further transmission. Ideally, the procedure should be delayed until adequate PPE is available, unless immediate action is the only viable option to save the patient's life.

Explanation:

Healthcare providers have an ethical duty to treat patients, but this duty is not absolute and must be weighed against the risk to their own safety and the potential for spreading infection to others. During infectious disease outbreaks, institutions have a reciprocal obligation to provide adequate protection and minimize risk. When such protection is lacking, physicians must consider alternative measures, such as delegating the procedure to a provider with available PPE, using modified airway techniques that reduce aerosolization, or employing telemedicine tools when possible. Ultimately, ethical decision-making should involve transparency, proportionality, and fairness, ensuring that neither patient care nor provider safety is unjustly compromised.

CHAPTER 12
End-of-Life Care and Palliative Sedation

Definition:

End-of-life care focuses on comfort, dignity, and quality of life for patients with terminal illnesses. Palliative sedation is the use of medications to reduce consciousness in order to relieve intractable and intolerable suffering that cannot be managed by other means at the end of life. It is ethically distinct from euthanasia, as the intent is to relieve suffering—not to hasten death.

Case Scenario (Ethical Dilemma):

Mr. Hale, a 66-year-old man with metastatic lung cancer, is in hospice and experiencing unbearable dyspnea and agitation despite maximal opioid therapy. He is fully aware and requests to be 'put to sleep permanently' due to his suffering. His family supports this request. The palliative team considers initiating palliative sedation but worries it may be seen as euthanasia.

Question:

Is initiating palliative sedation ethically appropriate in Mr. Hale's case? How can the team ensure it is ethically and legally justified?

Answer:

Yes, palliative sedation can be ethically appropriate if the suffering is refractory to other interventions, the intent is to relieve suffering (not to cause death), and informed consent is obtained.

Explanation:

Palliative sedation is a recognized part of ethical end-of-life care when symptoms are unrelieved by other means. Clear documentation of intent, informed consent, interdisciplinary consensus, and regular reassessment are essential. Unlike euthanasia, the primary goal is symptom relief, and it does not involve the deliberate act of ending life.

References:

- Canadian Society of Palliative Care Physicians (CSPCP): Guidelines on Palliative Sedation
- Canadian Medical Protective Association (CMPA): Palliative Sedation – Ethical and Legal Considerations
- CMA Code of Ethics and Professionalism
- College of Physicians and Surgeons of Ontario (CPSO): Planning for and Providing Quality End-of-Life Care

CHAPTER 13
Ethics of Experimental or Compassionate-Use Treatments

Definition:

Experimental treatments are medical interventions that have not yet received full regulatory approval and are often offered within the context of clinical trials. Compassionate-use treatments, also known as expanded access, involve providing investigational drugs or therapies to patients with serious or life-threatening conditions outside of clinical trials, typically when no comparable or satisfactory alternative therapy is available. These approaches raise complex ethical considerations regarding patient safety, informed consent, equity of access, and balancing hope with scientific rigor.

Case Scenario (Ethical Dilemma):

A 52-year-old patient with advanced pancreatic cancer has exhausted all approved treatment options. They have read about a promising investigational therapy that is in early-phase clinical trials overseas. The patient requests that you help them access the treatment through compassionate use. However, you are concerned about the lack of robust safety data, the high personal financial cost, and the possibility of exploitation by unregulated clinics. The patient's family is divided: some members support trying 'anything possible,' while others worry it may cause unnecessary suffering.

Question:

How should the physician ethically approach the patient's request for an experimental or compassionate-use treatment?

Answer:

The physician should engage in a thorough, balanced discussion with the patient, ensuring informed consent, evaluating the scientific validity of the treatment, confirming regulatory compliance, and considering the patient's values and quality-of-life goals before facilitating access.

Explanation:

Physicians must balance their duty to alleviate suffering with their responsibility to avoid harm. For experimental or compassionate-use treatments, this includes verifying the legitimacy of the intervention, its regulatory status, and any available safety and efficacy data. Informed consent is critical and must include discussion of uncertainties, potential benefits, risks, costs, and available alternatives. The physician should ensure the decision is free from coercion and aligns with the patient's values and goals of care. Where possible, treatments should be accessed through regulated pathways, such as Health Canada's Special Access Program, to ensure oversight, transparency, and protection of patient welfare.

CHAPTER 14
Genetic Testing and Privacy

Definition:

Genetic testing involves analyzing DNA to identify changes associated with inherited disorders or disease risk. Privacy in genetic testing is crucial due to the sensitive nature of the data, which may have implications not only for the individual but also for biological relatives. Healthcare providers must ensure informed consent, confidentiality, and appropriate use of genetic information.

Case Scenario (Ethical Dilemma):

Dr. Leung conducts genetic testing for a 35-year-old patient, Ms. N., and discovers she carries a BRCA1 mutation. Ms. N. refuses to inform her sister, who is also at risk. Dr. Leung worries that nondisclosure may place the sister in danger of undetected cancer risk but is unsure whether breaching confidentiality is ethically justifiable.

Question:

Can Dr. Leung ethically breach confidentiality to warn Ms. N.'s sister about the genetic risk?

Answer:

In most cases, confidentiality must be maintained. Breach is only considered if there is serious, foreseeable harm that can be prevented, and no alternative means to inform at-risk individuals.

Explanation:

Genetic information is protected under health privacy laws. While the potential harm to relatives may be significant, the ethical default is to respect patient confidentiality. Disclosure without consent may be considered only under strict conditions where risk is serious, imminent, and preventable. Physicians should counsel patients on the benefits of disclosure and offer genetic counselling support.

References:

- Canadian Medical Protective Association (CMPA): Genetic Testing and Privacy
- Personal Information Protection and Electronic Documents Act (PIPEDA)
- College of Physicians and Surgeons of Ontario (CPSO): Protecting Personal Health Information
- Canadian Medical Association (CMA) Code of Ethics and Professionalism
- Canadian Association of Genetic Counsellors (CAGC) Guidelines

CHAPTER 15
Global Health Ethics – Providing Care in Low-Resource Settings

Definition:

Global health ethics in low-resource settings addresses the moral principles, professional responsibilities, and decision-making frameworks guiding healthcare delivery in environments where infrastructure, staffing, and medical supplies are limited. Physicians must balance beneficence, justice, and respect for persons while navigating cultural, economic, and systemic challenges unique to such settings.

Case Scenario (Ethical Dilemma):

You are a physician volunteering in a rural clinic in a low-income country. The facility has only one ventilator, and two patients arrive simultaneously in respiratory failure—one is a young mother with pneumonia, and the other is an elderly man with advanced chronic lung disease. Local customs place a high value on elders, but clinical assessment suggests the younger patient has a better chance of survival. The community is closely observing your decision.

Question:

How should you approach the ethical decision-making process in allocating limited life-saving resources in a low-resource setting while respecting both medical ethics and local cultural values?

Answer:

Adopt a transparent, fair, and evidence-based triage process that prioritizes patients based on the likelihood of benefit and survival, while involving local healthcare leadership and respecting cultural norms. Communicate clearly with patients and families, and document the rationale for the decision to maintain trust.

Explanation:

Global health ethics emphasizes distributive justice, cultural humility, and resource stewardship. In low-resource settings, physicians must adapt triage frameworks—such as prioritizing patients with the greatest chance of recovery—to local realities. Transparent communication reduces mistrust, while engagement with local stakeholders ensures that decisions are culturally sensitive. The balance between medical utility and cultural respect is critical to maintaining ethical integrity and community trust.

CHAPTER 16
Informed Consent

Definition:

Informed consent is the process by which a healthcare provider discloses appropriate information to a competent patient so that the patient may make a voluntary choice to accept or refuse treatment. It is a foundational principle of medical ethics, grounded in respect for patient autonomy.

Case Scenario (Ethical Dilemma):

Dr. Ali is treating Mr. Thompson, a 72-year-old man recently diagnosed with a potentially operable brain tumor. Mr. Thompson's daughter, who is his caregiver, requests that Dr. Ali not disclose the diagnosis or the proposed neurosurgery to her father, fearing he will become depressed and refuse treatment. Mr. Thompson is mentally competent and has not indicated he does not wish to be informed. Dr. Ali is conflicted about whether respecting the daughter's wishes might violate informed consent requirements.

Question:

What is Dr. Ali's ethical obligation in this situation regarding informed consent?

Answer:

Dr. Ali is ethically obligated to disclose the diagnosis and treatment options to Mr. Thompson, as he is mentally competent and has not waived his right to be informed.

Explanation:

Informed consent requires that competent patients be provided with information necessary to make decisions about their own medical care. Unless a patient explicitly declines to receive such information, physicians are obligated to communicate honestly and completely. Family members cannot override a competent patient's right to know. Failure to disclose violates the ethical principles of autonomy and informed decision-making.

References:

- Canadian Medical Protective Association (CMPA): Consent – A Guide for Canadian Physicians
- College of Physicians and Surgeons of Ontario (CPSO): Informed Consent Policy
- Canadian Medical Association (CMA) Code of Ethics and Professionalism
- Beauchamp TL, Childress JF. Principles of Biomedical Ethics. 8th ed. Oxford University Press; 2019.

CHAPTER 17
Informed Consent in Pediatric Care – Parental vs. Child Decision Rights

Definition:

Informed consent in pediatric care involves obtaining permission for medical treatment from the appropriate decision-maker, balancing the legal authority of parents/guardians with the developing autonomy of the child. While parents generally have the legal right to consent for minors, mature minors may have the capacity to make certain decisions themselves. Ethical considerations include respecting the child's evolving capacity, protecting their welfare, and ensuring that decisions align with their best interests.

Case Scenario (Ethical Dilemma):

A 14-year-old boy presents to the rural emergency department with a forearm fracture sustained during a soccer match. He requires surgical fixation. The orthopedic surgeon explains the procedure and risks to both the boy and his parents. The child expresses strong refusal for surgery, fearing anesthesia, while both parents insist on proceeding, citing the long-term functional benefits. The care team must decide whose decision prevails.

Question:

In the context of informed consent for minors, how should the healthcare team proceed when the child refuses treatment but the parents consent?

Answer:

Assess the child's decision-making capacity using the mature minor standard. If the child demonstrates sufficient understanding of the procedure, risks, benefits, and alternatives, their refusal may carry legal and ethical weight. If capacity is lacking, parental consent generally prevails. Engage in shared decision-making, provide additional counseling, and involve child advocacy services if needed.

Explanation:

Canadian law recognizes the concept of the 'mature minor,' which allows a minor with sufficient maturity to make their own healthcare decisions. Capacity is based on the individual's ability to understand relevant information and appreciate the consequences of their decision. In practice, most jurisdictions prioritize the best interests of the child while considering their autonomy. If the child is deemed capable, their informed refusal must be respected unless it poses a serious threat to life or health. In cases of disagreement, mediation and ethics consultation are recommended. In rural settings, where access to such resources may be limited, clear communication, empathy, and documentation of the consent process are essential.

CHAPTER 18
Mandatory Reporting (e.g., Child Abuse, Elder Abuse)

Definition:

Mandatory reporting refers to the legal obligation of healthcare providers to report certain types of suspected harm, such as child abuse, elder abuse, or neglect, to the appropriate authorities. This duty overrides patient confidentiality and is designed to protect vulnerable individuals from harm.

Case Scenario (Ethical Dilemma):

Dr. Chen evaluates an 82-year-old woman who presents with bruises, poor hygiene, and vague explanations about her injuries. She lives with her adult son, who answers most questions and insists everything is fine. The patient quietly denies abuse but appears fearful. Dr. Chen is uncertain whether to report her suspicions without the patient's consent.

Question:

Is Dr. Chen legally and ethically required to report this suspected elder abuse, even if the patient does not confirm it?

Answer:

Yes. Healthcare providers are legally required to report suspected abuse of vulnerable individuals, even without the patient's confirmation or consent.

Explanation:

Mandatory reporting laws prioritize protection of at-risk individuals. In cases of suspected abuse or neglect, physicians must report their concerns to designated authorities. Patient confidentiality is overridden by this legal duty. Reports must be made in good faith based on reasonable suspicion, not conclusive proof. Failure to report may result in harm and legal consequences.

References:

- Child and Family Services Act (Ontario), 1990
- Canadian Medical Protective Association (CMPA): Mandatory Reporting Guidelines
- College of Physicians and Surgeons of Ontario (CPSO): Reporting Obligations Policy
- Canadian Medical Association (CMA) Code of Ethics and Professionalism

CHAPTER 19
Managing Medical Errors and Disclosure

Definition:

Managing medical errors ethically involves promptly recognizing, disclosing, and addressing adverse events or near misses that occur in patient care. Disclosure requires honest communication, acknowledgment of the event, an explanation of what happened, and a plan to prevent recurrence. It supports patient trust, transparency, and learning within the healthcare system.

Case Scenario (Ethical Dilemma):

A nurse informs Dr. Taylor that the wrong antibiotic dose was given to a patient, Mr. R., who has now developed acute kidney injury. Dr. Taylor is unsure how much detail to provide to Mr. R. and his family, especially since the prognosis is uncertain and fear of legal consequences looms among staff.

Question:

What are Dr. Taylor's ethical responsibilities in disclosing the medical error to the patient and family?

Answer:

Dr. Taylor must fully disclose the error, express empathy, explain known and unknown factors, and initiate a plan for follow-up and safety improvement.

Explanation:

Ethical and professional standards mandate open disclosure of medical errors. Patients have the right to know what occurred, especially if harm resulted. A respectful and transparent conversation includes acknowledgment, regret or apology, and efforts to learn from the event. Institutions must foster a culture of safety, not blame, to support ethical responses and systemic improvement.

References:

- Canadian Medical Protective Association (CMPA): Disclosing Harm from Healthcare Delivery
- Canadian Medical Association (CMA) Code of Ethics and Professionalism
- Institute for Safe Medication Practices Canada (ISMP): Disclosure Guidelines
- College of Physicians and Surgeons of Ontario (CPSO): Disclosure of Harm Policy

CHAPTER 20
Medical Assistance in Dying (MAiD)

Definition:

Medical Assistance in Dying (MAiD) refers to the legally sanctioned process by which a physician or nurse practitioner provides or administers medication that intentionally brings about a patient's death, at the patient's voluntary and competent request. In Canada, MAiD is governed by federal and provincial legislation and is subject to strict eligibility criteria and safeguards.

Case Scenario (Ethical Dilemma):

Ms. Dupuis, a 62-year-old woman with metastatic breast cancer, requests MAiD due to progressive pain and loss of dignity. Her physician, Dr. Norris, has a conscientious objection to MAiD and feels deeply uncomfortable facilitating or referring for the procedure. Ms. Dupuis is distressed and insists on her right to access MAiD without delay.

Question:

What are Dr. Norris's ethical obligations in this scenario, and how should he respond to Ms. Dupuis's request?

Answer:

Dr. Norris is ethically and legally required to ensure Ms. Dupuis has timely access to MAiD, even if he objects to participating. He must make an effective referral to another provider or institution.

Explanation:

While healthcare professionals may conscientiously object to MAiD, they cannot obstruct patient access to legal medical services. In jurisdictions like Ontario, physicians are required to provide an effective referral. This balances the provider's right to conscience with the patient's right to access care. Clear documentation, compassionate communication, and timely referral are key ethical duties.

References:

- Government of Canada: MAiD Legislation and Criteria
- Canadian Medical Protective Association (CMPA): MAiD and the Role of Physicians
- College of Physicians and Surgeons of Ontario (CPSO): MAiD Policy
- Canadian Medical Association (CMA) Policy on Medical Assistance in Dying

CHAPTER 21
Patient Refusal of Treatment

Definition:

Patient refusal of treatment refers to a competent individual's right to decline medical interventions, even if the decision may lead to harm or death. This principle is grounded in respect for autonomy. Physicians must ensure the patient is informed, capable, and not under coercion when refusing care.

Case Scenario (Ethical Dilemma):

Mr. L, a 52-year-old man with poorly controlled type 1 diabetes, is admitted with severe sepsis and is advised to undergo urgent surgery to drain an infected abscess. He refuses surgery, stating he is tired of interventions and prefers to 'let nature take its course.' His family pleads with the team to convince him otherwise. The attending physician is concerned about the risk of death if treatment is not provided.

Question:

Can the healthcare team proceed with surgery against Mr. L's wishes if he is deemed capable of making this decision?

Answer:

No. If Mr. L is capable and fully informed, his decision must be respected, even if it may result in death.

Explanation:

Capable patients have the legal and ethical right to refuse any medical treatment. The physician's role is to ensure the patient understands the nature, risks, and consequences of refusal. If Mr. L is found competent and the decision is voluntary and informed, it must be honored. Physicians should offer emotional support, explore concerns, and document the discussion thoroughly.

References:

- Health Care Consent Act (Ontario), 1996
- Canadian Medical Protective Association (CMPA): When Patients Refuse Treatment
- College of Physicians and Surgeons of Ontario (CPSO): Consent to Treatment Policy
- Canadian Medical Association (CMA) Code of Ethics and Professionalism

CHAPTER 22
Physician-Assisted Suicide vs. Euthanasia Distinctions

Definition:

Physician-assisted suicide (PAS) involves a physician providing a patient with the means to end their own life, usually through a prescribed lethal medication. Euthanasia involves the physician directly administering a substance to intentionally end the patient's life. In Canada, both are encompassed under Medical Assistance in Dying (MAiD), but the ethical and procedural distinctions remain important.

Case Scenario (Ethical Dilemma):

Ms. R., a 59-year-old with terminal ALS, requests Medical Assistance in Dying. She is physically unable to self-administer the medication and asks Dr. Jones to proceed with euthanasia. Dr. Jones is comfortable with assisted suicide but personally objects to administering the lethal dose. He wonders whether referring the case constitutes moral participation in euthanasia.

Question:

What are Dr. Jones's ethical obligations in this situation, and how should he navigate the distinction between PAS and euthanasia?

Answer:

Dr. Jones may decline to perform euthanasia due to conscientious objection but is ethically obligated to provide an effective referral to support the patient's legal right to access care.

Explanation:

While PAS and euthanasia differ in physician involvement, the ethical obligation to ensure patient access to care remains. In jurisdictions where both practices are legal (like Canada under MAiD), physicians must follow legal safeguards and uphold patient autonomy, even if they do not personally participate. Providing an effective referral maintains the balance between professional conscience and patient rights.

References:

- Government of Canada: Medical Assistance in Dying (MAiD) Legislation
- Canadian Medical Association (CMA): MAiD Policy and Ethics
- Canadian Medical Protective Association (CMPA): Ethics of MAiD and Conscientious Objection
- College of Physicians and Surgeons of Ontario (CPSO): MAiD Policy and Referral Obligations

CHAPTER 23
Physician Conscientious Objection

Definition:

Conscientious objection occurs when a physician refuses to provide or participate in certain medical services due to deeply held moral, ethical, or religious beliefs. While physicians have a right to moral integrity, they also have a duty to respect patient autonomy and ensure access to legally available medical care.

Case Scenario (Ethical Dilemma):

Dr. Morgan, a family physician, is approached by a long-time patient requesting a referral for abortion services. Dr. Morgan has a conscientious objection to abortion and feels morally unable to participate. The patient is upset, stating she expected compassionate help, not judgment.

Question:

Can Dr. Morgan ethically refuse to provide or refer for abortion services based on personal beliefs?

Answer:

Dr. Morgan may decline to participate due to conscientious objection but is ethically and legally required to provide an effective referral to another provider.

Explanation:

Conscientious objection is recognized in medical ethics, but it does not allow physicians to abandon patients or obstruct access to care. In Ontario and other jurisdictions, physicians must provide an effective referral to ensure timely access to legal services. Respectful communication, documentation, and nondiscriminatory care are essential.

References:

- College of Physicians and Surgeons of Ontario (CPSO): Professional Obligations and Human Rights Policy
- Canadian Medical Association (CMA) Code of Ethics and Professionalism
- Canadian Medical Protective Association (CMPA): Conscientious Objection Guidance
- Carter v. Canada, 2015 SCC 5 – Legal Context for MAiD and Objection

CHAPTER 24
Privacy Breaches and Data Security

Definition:

Privacy breaches in healthcare involve unauthorized access, disclosure, or loss of personal health information. Data security refers to the technical and organizational measures used to protect this information from breaches. Healthcare professionals and institutions are ethically and legally responsible for safeguarding patient information and responding appropriately to any breach.

Case Scenario (Ethical Dilemma):

Dr. Singh accidentally sends a diagnostic report containing personal health information to the wrong patient by email. Upon realizing the error, she deletes the message and hesitates to report the incident, thinking it caused no visible harm and may damage her professional standing.

Question:

What are Dr. Singh's ethical and legal responsibilities after a privacy breach, even if the impact seems minimal?

Answer:

Dr. Singh must report the breach to the appropriate privacy officer, document the event, notify the affected patient, and take corrective steps to prevent recurrence.

Explanation:

Privacy and confidentiality are core to patient trust. Even unintentional breaches must be acknowledged and managed transparently. Legal frameworks such as PHIPA (Ontario) mandate disclosure and documentation. Failing to report breaches can compound harm and erode trust. Education, secure communication tools, and privacy audits reduce future risks.

References

This reference list includes publicly available legal and ethical guidelines from Canadian regulatory and professional bodies. These sources were consulted for general ethical principles in healthcare. No proprietary or restricted material has been reproduced. All references are accessible to the public and used in accordance with fair use for educational purposes.

- Personal Health Information Protection Act (PHIPA), Ontario
- Canadian Medical Protective Association (CMPA): Managing Privacy Breaches
- College of Physicians and Surgeons of Ontario (CPSO): Protecting Personal Health Information
- Canadian Medical Association (CMA) Code of Ethics and Professionalism

CHAPTER 25
Professional Boundaries

Definition:

Professional boundaries refer to the limits that define the appropriate interactions and roles between healthcare providers and patients. Maintaining these boundaries is essential to preserve trust, objectivity, and the integrity of the physician–patient relationship.

Case Scenario (Ethical Dilemma):

Dr. Malik has been seeing Ms. A, a 28-year-old patient, for several years to manage her chronic migraines. They have developed a rapport, and after a recent visit, Ms. A asks Dr. Malik if he would like to have coffee with her socially. Dr. Malik is flattered but unsure whether accepting would cross a professional line.

Question:

Should Dr. Malik accept the invitation for coffee with his patient?

Answer:

No. Accepting the invitation risks crossing professional boundaries and may compromise the therapeutic relationship.

Explanation:

Physicians must maintain clear professional boundaries to avoid conflicts of interest, emotional entanglement, and exploitation. Even seemingly innocent social interactions can blur roles and lead to ethical complications. Dr. Malik should politely decline and explain that maintaining professional distance is in the best interest of the patient–physician relationship.

References:

- Canadian Medical Association (CMA) Code of Ethics and Professionalism
- Canadian Medical Protective Association (CMPA): Maintaining Appropriate Boundaries
- College of Physicians and Surgeons of Ontario (CPSO): Boundary Violations Policy
- Federation of Medical Regulatory Authorities of Canada (FMRAC): Guidelines on Professionalism

CHAPTER 26
Research Ethics and Human Subjects Protection

Definition:

Research ethics involves applying moral principles to the planning, conduct, and reporting of research involving human participants. Human subjects protection ensures participants' rights, safety, and well-being are prioritized through informed consent, risk minimization, confidentiality, and ethical oversight by research ethics boards (REBs).

Case Scenario (Ethical Dilemma):

Dr. Nguyen is conducting a clinical study on a new antihypertensive drug in a low-income community. Some participants struggle to understand the complex consent forms. A few appear to enroll primarily for the free check-ups and transportation. A colleague raises concern that participants may not fully grasp the risks or their right to withdraw. Dr. Nguyen is unsure whether the study's consent process is adequate.

Question:

How should Dr. Nguyen respond to concerns about informed consent and participant understanding in the study?

Answer:

Dr. Nguyen must ensure that all participants provide truly informed consent. The study process should be revised to enhance comprehension and protect participant autonomy.

Explanation:

Informed consent must be voluntary, informed, and comprehensible to participants. Researchers must avoid exploiting vulnerable populations and ensure that consent is not influenced by undue inducement. REBs play a key role in monitoring study protocols and consent practices. Ethics in research demands prioritizing participant welfare over scientific goals.

References:

- Tri-Council Policy Statement: Ethical Conduct for Research Involving Humans (TCPS 2, Canada)
- Canadian Medical Association (CMA) Code of Ethics and Professionalism
- World Medical Association Declaration of Helsinki
- Canadian Institutes of Health Research (CIHR): Human Ethics Guidelines

CHAPTER 27
Reporting Impaired or Incompetent Colleagues

Definition:

Healthcare professionals have an ethical and legal duty to report colleagues whose physical or mental health, or professional behavior, poses a risk to patient safety. This includes impairment from substance use, mental illness, or incompetence due to lack of knowledge or skill. Reporting must be done in good faith, with patient safety as the primary concern.

Case Scenario (Ethical Dilemma):

Dr. James notices that his colleague, Dr. R, has been frequently disoriented during rounds, forgetting patient names and orders, and smelling of alcohol. Several nurses have expressed concern, but no one has taken formal action. Dr. James is conflicted—he doesn't want to betray a colleague but worries about patient harm.

Question:

What is Dr. James's ethical obligation in this situation, and how should he proceed?

Answer:

Dr. James has a duty to report the situation to the appropriate regulatory or hospital authority to protect patients and support Dr. R's recovery.

Explanation:

Patient safety must take precedence over professional loyalty. Physicians have a duty to report impaired or incompetent colleagues to their regulatory body or hospital leadership. Early intervention may allow impaired colleagues to receive support or rehabilitation. Failure to act may result in patient harm and legal or professional consequences for the witness.

References:

- Canadian Medical Protective Association (CMPA): Duty to Report Colleagues
- College of Physicians and Surgeons of Ontario (CPSO): Mandatory and Permissive Reporting
- Canadian Medical Association (CMA) Code of Ethics and Professionalism
- Health Professions Procedural Code, Regulated Health Professions Act (Ontario)

CHAPTER 28
Sexual Harassment and Discrimination

Definition:

Sexual harassment includes unwelcome sexual advances, comments, or conduct that creates an intimidating or hostile environment. Discrimination in healthcare refers to unfair treatment based on gender, race, ethnicity, sexual orientation, disability, or other protected characteristics. Both are serious violations of ethical and professional standards.

Case Scenario (Ethical Dilemma):

Dr. Ali, a female resident, reports that a senior attending physician made repeated inappropriate comments about her appearance during clinical rounds. Other team members witnessed the behavior but dismissed it as 'harmless jokes.' Dr. Ali feels uncomfortable and unsupported but fears retaliation if she formally complains.

Question:

What are the ethical and institutional responsibilities in this case, and how should the situation be addressed?

Answer:

The behavior constitutes sexual harassment and must be reported to the institution's appropriate body. There is an ethical and legal duty to support a safe, respectful work environment.

Explanation:

Sexual harassment and discrimination undermine trust, professional integrity, and psychological safety. Institutions must provide clear reporting mechanisms, protect whistleblowers from retaliation, and act promptly. Bystanders have a duty to support affected individuals.

Medical professionals must uphold respect and equity as part of ethical practice.

References:

- Canadian Medical Association (CMA) Policy on Equity and Diversity in Medicine
- Canadian Medical Protective Association (CMPA): Responding to Harassment
- College of Physicians and Surgeons of Ontario (CPSO): Professional Conduct Policies
- Ontario Human Rights Code
- University Health Network: Code of Conduct and Anti-Harassment Guidelines

CHAPTER 29
Social Media Use by Physicians – Boundaries and Professional Image

Definition:

Social media use by physicians encompasses the creation, sharing, and interaction with online content across platforms such as Facebook, Twitter (X), Instagram, LinkedIn, and medical forums. While these tools can enhance professional communication, networking, and patient education, they also present risks to confidentiality, professional boundaries, and public trust. Physicians must balance personal expression with their ethical and professional obligations.

Case Scenario (Ethical Dilemma):

Dr. Ahmed, a family physician in a small rural community, posts a photo on Instagram from a community charity event. In the background, a patient can be identified wearing a hospital gown. Later, a colleague mentions that the post could be considered a privacy breach, even though the patient's name was not mentioned. The post is quickly gaining attention online.

Question:

What ethical issues should Dr. Ahmed consider before posting on social media, and what steps should be taken to maintain professional boundaries and protect patient privacy?

Answer:

- Remove the post immediately to prevent further dissemination.
- Acknowledge and reflect on the privacy breach.
- Seek guidance from institutional or regulatory policies on social media use.

- Implement stricter personal rules for reviewing content before posting.
- Educate colleagues and staff on safe social media practices.

Explanation:

Physicians have a duty to protect patient confidentiality both in clinical and non-clinical contexts. Even unintentional identification of patients in social media posts may constitute a privacy breach under Canadian privacy laws (e.g., PHIPA, HIPA). Professional boundaries can also be blurred when personal and professional personas overlap online. Maintaining a separate professional account, using strict privacy settings, and avoiding sharing patient-related content without explicit, documented consent are key strategies. Regulatory bodies encourage transparency, professionalism, and caution in all online interactions to preserve public trust in the medical profession.

CHAPTER 30
Stigmatization and Discrimination in Healthcare

Definition:

Stigmatization and discrimination in healthcare refer to negative attitudes, behaviors, or systemic practices that unfairly target individuals based on characteristics such as race, gender, mental illness, substance use, disability, or socioeconomic status. These actions undermine equity, quality of care, and the patient–provider relationship.

Case Scenario (Ethical Dilemma):

Mr. T., a 38-year-old man with a history of opioid use disorder, presents to the emergency department with abdominal pain. The triage nurse comments that he's likely drug-seeking and places him lower on the triage priority list. A junior physician later identifies acute appendicitis, requiring urgent surgery. Mr. T. expresses concern that he is treated differently every time he visits the hospital.

Question:

What are the ethical responsibilities of healthcare providers in addressing stigma and ensuring equitable care for all patients?

Answer:

Healthcare providers must recognize and actively work to eliminate bias and discrimination. All patients deserve respectful, evidence-based, and equitable care regardless of background or history.

Explanation:

Stigma undermines the ethical principles of justice, non-maleficence, and respect for persons. Providers must reflect on personal biases, avoid assumptions, and follow clinical guidelines in an unbiased manner. Institutions should implement anti-stigma training and create inclusive environments. Failure to address discrimination leads to health disparities and loss of patient trust.

References:

- Canadian Medical Association (CMA) Policy on Equity and Diversity in Medicine
- Canadian Human Rights Act
- Canadian Medical Protective Association (CMPA): Stigma and Patient Safety
- Ontario Human Rights Commission: Policy on Discrimination in Healthcare

CHAPTER 31
Surrogate Decision-Making

Definition:

Surrogate decision-making occurs when someone makes healthcare decisions on behalf of a patient who lacks the capacity to decide for themselves. The surrogate is expected to follow the patient's known wishes or, if unknown, act in the patient's best interests. Surrogates may be legally appointed or designated through prior directive.

Case Scenario (Ethical Dilemma):

Mrs. K, a 79-year-old woman with advanced dementia, is hospitalized with severe pneumonia. She lacks decision-making capacity and has no advance directive. Her daughter, the substitute decision-maker, requests full intensive care, including intubation. The medical team believes aggressive treatment would be non-beneficial and cause unnecessary suffering.

Question:

How should the healthcare team approach this disagreement with the surrogate regarding the intensity of care?

Answer:

The team should engage in clear communication, explain the medical futility, and, if needed, consult ethics or legal services to resolve the conflict in line with best interest standards.

Explanation:

Surrogates must act in accordance with the patient's known values and preferences, or otherwise in the patient's best interests. When requested care is likely to cause harm without meaningful benefit, the care team is not ethically obligated to provide it. Facilitated discussion, palliative consultation, or hospital ethics support may help resolve disagreements while respecting the patient's dignity and minimizing suffering.

References:

- Health Care Consent Act (Ontario), 1996
- Canadian Medical Protective Association (CMPA): Substitute Decision-Making
- College of Physicians and Surgeons of Ontario (CPSO): Planning and Providing End-of-Life Care
- Canadian Medical Association (CMA) Code of Ethics and Professionalism

CHAPTER 32
Telemedicine and Digital Health Ethics

Definition:

Telemedicine and digital health involve providing healthcare services and consultations using digital platforms, such as video calls, apps, and electronic communications. Ethical considerations include privacy, confidentiality, quality of care, informed consent, equity in access, and maintaining the patient–provider relationship.

Case Scenario (Ethical Dilemma):

Dr. Silva conducts a virtual follow-up with a patient who lives in a rural area. The internet connection is poor, making it difficult to assess a new skin lesion the patient describes as growing and painful. The patient declines an in-person visit due to travel costs. Dr. Silva is unsure whether to prescribe treatment without a proper visual exam.

Question:

What are Dr. Silva's ethical obligations in balancing access to care with the need for a proper clinical assessment?

Answer:

Dr. Silva must ensure clinical decisions meet the standard of care. If the quality of assessment is inadequate, she must recommend in-person follow-up or referral.

Explanation:

Telemedicine must meet the same ethical and clinical standards as in-person care. When virtual limitations compromise assessment, the provider must take steps to avoid misdiagnosis or harm. Clinicians must document limitations, advise appropriate follow-up, and ensure informed consent specific to virtual care, including risks and limitations.

References:

- Canadian Medical Association (CMA) Policy on Telemedicine
- College of Physicians and Surgeons of Ontario (CPSO): Virtual Care Policy
- Canadian Medical Protective Association (CMPA): Legal and Ethical Considerations in Digital Health
- Canadian Institute for Health Information (CIHI): Virtual Care Use in Canada

CHAPTER 33
Truth-telling vs. Therapeutic Privilege

Definition:

Truth-telling is the ethical obligation of healthcare providers to be honest and transparent with patients about their diagnosis, prognosis, and treatment options. Therapeutic privilege refers to the rare exception where disclosure of information is withheld because it is believed that full disclosure would cause serious harm to the patient's physical or mental health.

Case Scenario (Ethical Dilemma):

Dr. Bennett is treating Mr. Costa, a 76-year-old man recently diagnosed with terminal pancreatic cancer. Mr. Costa has a history of severe depression. His wife pleads with Dr. Bennett not to reveal the diagnosis, fearing it would drive him into a suicidal crisis. Dr. Bennett wonders whether withholding the diagnosis might be ethically permissible under therapeutic privilege.

Question:

Is Dr. Bennett justified in withholding the diagnosis under therapeutic privilege?

Answer:

Not unless there is compelling, evidence-based concern that disclosure would cause serious and imminent harm. Therapeutic privilege should be used only in exceptional cases.

Explanation:

While protecting patients from harm is an ethical responsibility, overriding the principle of autonomy through therapeutic privilege is rarely justified. Dr. Bennett must assess Mr. Costa's mental health status, consider involving psychiatry, and explore ways to deliver the information sensitively. Truth-telling can be tempered with compassion and timing, but withholding essential health information violates informed consent and risks damaging trust.

References:

- Canadian Medical Protective Association (CMPA): Truth-telling and Therapeutic Privilege
- Canadian Medical Association (CMA) Code of Ethics and Professionalism
- College of Physicians and Surgeons of Ontario (CPSO): Consent and Disclosure
- Beauchamp TL, Childress JF. Principles of Biomedical Ethics. 8th ed. Oxford University Press; 2019.

CHAPTER 34
Use of Restraints (Physical and Chemical)

Definition:

Restraints refer to methods used to restrict a patient's movement or behavior. Physical restraints include devices like wrist ties or bed rails, while chemical restraints involve sedative medications given to control behavior. The use of restraints must follow ethical and legal standards, prioritizing patient dignity, safety, and the least restrictive means necessary.

Case Scenario (Ethical Dilemma):

Mr. J., a 76-year-old man with delirium, repeatedly attempts to get out of bed and pull out his IV line despite being at high risk of falling. The night nurse applies wrist restraints without a physician's order, intending to prevent injury. In the morning, Mr. J. is confused, bruised, and distressed. His daughter demands an explanation.

Question:

Was the application of restraints justified in this case? What are the ethical obligations regarding restraint use?

Answer:

No. Restraints should only be used as a last resort with proper assessment, physician involvement, consent when feasible, and regular monitoring.

Explanation:

The use of restraints without appropriate indication, documentation, or physician oversight can violate patient rights and cause harm. Ethical care requires exploring alternatives like reorientation, supervision, or low beds. If restraints are used, clear justification, time-limited use, and ongoing evaluation are essential. Staff must follow institutional policies and prioritize the patient's dignity and safety.

References:

- Canadian Medical Protective Association (CMPA): Use of Restraints in Healthcare
- Canadian Patient Safety Institute (CPSI): Least Restraint Policy
- College of Physicians and Surgeons of Ontario (CPSO): Responsibilities in Use of Restraints
- Canadian Nurses Association (CNA): Code of Ethics – Restraint Use

CHAPTER 35
Whistleblowing – Ethical and Legal Protections for Healthcare Providers

Definition:

Whistleblowing in healthcare refers to the act of reporting unethical, illegal, or unsafe practices within a healthcare setting to internal or external authorities. This may involve exposing patient safety risks, fraud, abuse, or violations of professional and legal obligations. Ethical whistleblowing balances the duty to protect patients and uphold professional standards against potential personal and professional risks to the whistleblower.

Case Scenario (Ethical Dilemma):

A registered nurse in a rural hospital discovers that a senior physician has been falsifying patient records to cover up repeated medication errors. The nurse reports the issue internally to hospital administration, but no action is taken. She is now considering reporting the matter to the provincial regulatory authority but fears retaliation, job loss, and damage to her reputation.

Question:

What are the ethical and legal considerations for the nurse when deciding whether to escalate her report to an external authority?

Answer:

The nurse must weigh her ethical duty to protect patients and uphold professional integrity against potential personal consequences. She should follow established internal reporting channels first, document her concerns, and ensure that all communication is factual and evidence-based. If internal avenues fail to address the problem, she has an ethical and, in many cases, a legal obligation to report externally to the relevant regulatory or oversight bodies. Legal protections for whistleblowers may exist under provincial or federal legislation, but these vary by jurisdiction.

Explanation:

Whistleblowing in healthcare is justified when patient safety, public trust, or the integrity of the profession is at risk. Ethical principles such as beneficence, non-maleficence, and justice support taking action to prevent harm. However, the decision is often complicated by fears of retaliation or professional isolation. Healthcare providers should be familiar with their institution's policies, professional codes of ethics, and applicable whistleblower protection laws. In Canada, some provinces have specific whistleblower protection acts for healthcare workers, while others rely on broader employment and human rights legislation.

CHAPTER 36
Withdrawal or Withholding of Life-Sustaining Treatment

Definition:

Withholding life-sustaining treatment refers to the decision not to initiate a potentially life-prolonging intervention (e.g., mechanical ventilation, dialysis). Withdrawal refers to the discontinuation of an ongoing intervention. Both are ethically and legally acceptable when treatment is deemed non-beneficial or contrary to a patient's wishes or best interests.

Case Scenario (Ethical Dilemma):

Mrs. Patel, a 70-year-old woman with end-stage heart failure, is admitted to the ICU with respiratory failure. She is intubated and started on inotropes. Despite maximal therapy, her condition deteriorates. Her advance directive declines life-prolonging treatment in terminal illness. Her family insists on continuing aggressive measures, saying she was 'always a fighter' and might recover.

Question:

Is it ethically justifiable to withdraw life-sustaining treatments in this case, even if the family disagrees?

Answer:

Yes. If the patient's condition is irreversible and her advance directive is clear, continuing aggressive treatment would violate her wishes. Withdrawal is ethically justified.

Explanation:

When a valid advance directive exists and the clinical team determines that further intervention is non-beneficial, they are ethically obligated to align care with the patient's expressed values. Withdrawal of treatment is not equivalent to euthanasia—it allows the natural course of the illness to proceed. While families should be supported and heard, their disagreement does not override the patient's autonomy or clinical judgment.

References:

- Canadian Medical Protective Association (CMPA): Withholding and Withdrawing Life-Sustaining Treatment
- College of Physicians and Surgeons of Ontario (CPSO): Planning for and Providing Quality End-of-Life Care
- Canadian Medical Association (CMA) Code of Ethics and Professionalism
- Downar J, et al. Ethical considerations in the withdrawal of life-sustaining therapies. Can J Gen Intern Med. 2017.

CHAPTER 37
Workplace Bullying and Professional Respect in Healthcare Teams

Definition:

Workplace bullying in healthcare refers to repeated, health-harming mistreatment of one or more individuals by one or more perpetrators. It may include verbal abuse, offensive conduct/behaviors (including nonverbal), and work interference that undermines a colleague's ability to perform their role. Professional respect involves maintaining dignity, fairness, and collaboration among healthcare team members, ensuring safe patient care and a supportive work environment.

Case Scenario (Ethical Dilemma):

Dr. Ahmed, a junior physician, notices that one of the senior consultants frequently belittles and excludes a nurse from important ward discussions. The nurse has become withdrawn, is taking more sick days, and her performance is being questioned by other staff. Dr. Ahmed is unsure whether to report the behavior, fearing retaliation and damage to his working relationships.

Question:

What should Dr. Ahmed do to address the situation while maintaining professionalism and protecting patient safety?

Answer:

Dr. Ahmed should document the incidents, support the affected colleague, and report the bullying behavior through the institution's formal reporting channels or human resources. He should encourage a respectful dialogue when possible and ensure that patient safety is prioritized by addressing the toxic behavior.

Explanation:

Workplace bullying undermines teamwork, morale, and patient safety. Ethical principles require healthcare professionals to foster respectful, supportive environments. Addressing bullying is a professional duty and often a regulatory requirement. Institutions should have clear anti-bullying policies, confidential reporting systems, and support mechanisms. Failure to address such behavior can lead to burnout, errors, and high staff turnover. While fear of retaliation is a legitimate concern, proper documentation, adherence to reporting protocols, and involving trusted supervisors or mentors can help protect whistleblowers.

CLINICAL SCENARIOS

Access to Care and Health Equity

Scenario: A low-income patient cannot afford transportation to the hospital for regular dialysis.

Question: What ethical principle is most relevant here?

Answer: Justice — ensuring equitable access to healthcare resources.

Explanation: Physicians and systems have an ethical duty to minimize barriers to care, advocate for resources, and address social determinants of health.

Advance Directives and Goals of Care

Scenario: A patient's advance directive states 'Do not intubate.' He arrives in the ER with severe pneumonia and respiratory failure.

Question: Should the healthcare team proceed with intubation?

Answer: No.

Explanation: Advance directives express a patient's wishes when they cannot communicate. Respecting these instructions is essential to uphold patient autonomy and legal requirements.

Allocation of Scarce Resources (e.g., ICU beds, transplant organs)

Scenario: During a pandemic, ICU beds are limited, and two critically ill patients require admission.

Question: What is the ethical approach to deciding who receives the ICU bed?

Answer: Apply transparent, fair, and evidence-based triage criteria established by institutional or public health policies.

Explanation: Allocation decisions should be based on maximizing benefit, fairness, and consistency, avoiding bias or preferential treatment. Ethical frameworks help ensure trust in the process.

Artificial Intelligence and Decision Support in Medicine – Ethical Considerations

Scenario: A hospital introduces an AI tool to help diagnose rare conditions. A physician receives an AI recommendation that conflicts with their clinical judgment.

Question: How should the physician proceed when AI recommendations conflict with clinical expertise?

Answer: The physician should prioritize patient safety, use AI as a supportive tool, and base the final decision on clinical judgment while documenting reasoning.

Explanation: AI can enhance diagnostic accuracy but must not override human judgment. Physicians are ethically obligated to validate AI suggestions and ensure decisions align with best practices and patient values.

Breaking Bad News

Scenario: A patient's biopsy results confirm metastatic cancer. The family asks the physician to avoid telling the patient to 'protect' them.

Question: Should the physician withhold the diagnosis from the patient?

Answer: No, unless the patient has clearly expressed a wish not to know.

Explanation: Patients have the right to know their diagnosis and prognosis. Information should be delivered with empathy, ensuring support is available.

Capacity and Decision-Making

Scenario: A 78-year-old with early dementia insists on refusing a life-saving blood transfusion. She can explain her choice and the consequences clearly.

Question: Does this patient have decision-making capacity?

Answer: Yes.

Explanation: Capacity is task-specific and requires understanding, appreciation, reasoning, and expression of choice. Despite dementia, she demonstrates adequate capacity for this decision.

Confidentiality and Privacy

Scenario: A teenage patient is diagnosed with a sexually transmitted infection. Her parent calls asking for details about her visit.

Question: Should the physician disclose the diagnosis to the parent without the patient's consent?

Answer: No, unless disclosure is legally required.

Explanation: Physicians must protect patient confidentiality, even for minors, unless there is a clear legal obligation to disclose or imminent risk to the patient or others.

Conflict of Interest

Scenario: A physician is invited to speak at a conference sponsored by a pharmaceutical company whose drug they frequently prescribe.

Question: What should the physician do to manage potential conflict of interest?

Answer: Disclose the relationship and ensure content is evidence-based.

Explanation: Transparency about financial or professional ties helps maintain trust and reduces bias. The physician must ensure recommendations are based on best evidence, not sponsor influence.

Cultural Sensitivity and Respect for Indigenous Health Practices

Scenario: A patient from an Indigenous community prefers traditional healing methods over hospital-based treatments for a chronic condition.

Question: How should the physician approach this situation?

Answer: Engage in respectful dialogue, explore the patient's preferences, and collaborate to integrate safe traditional practices with evidence-based care.

Explanation: Respecting cultural practices builds trust and improves adherence to care. The physician should avoid dismissing the patient's beliefs and instead find ways to align medical treatment with cultural values.

Do Not Resuscitate (DNR) Orders

Scenario: A 78-year-old patient with advanced heart failure is admitted with pneumonia. His family insists on full resuscitation despite the patient's documented DNR order.

Question: How should the physician proceed?

Answer: Honor the patient's documented DNR order.

Explanation: A valid DNR order reflects the patient's autonomous decision and must be respected. Family wishes cannot override a competent patient's documented choice unless legal grounds invalidate the order.

Duty to Treat vs. Physician Safety During Infectious Disease Outbreaks

Scenario: Scenario: During an Ebola outbreak, a physician is asked to treat infected patients but fears for their own safety due to limited protective equipment.

Question: Question: What factors should guide the physician's decision?

Answer: Balance the duty to care with the obligation to minimize personal risk.

Explanation: Explanation: Physicians have a professional duty to treat patients but are not obligated to take unreasonable personal risks. Adequate PPE and institutional safety measures should be in place before providing care.

End-of-Life Care and Palliative Sedation

Scenario: A 68-year-old woman with advanced pancreatic cancer is experiencing intractable pain and agitation despite optimized analgesia. The palliative care team suggests palliative sedation to relieve suffering.

Question: Is it ethically acceptable to initiate palliative sedation in this case?

Answer: Yes, when symptoms are refractory and the intent is comfort, not hastening death.

Explanation: Palliative sedation is ethically acceptable if it is intended to relieve intolerable symptoms in a terminally ill patient, with informed consent obtained from the patient or substitute decision-maker.

Ethics of Experimental or Compassionate-Use Treatments

Scenario: A patient with a terminal illness requests access to an unapproved experimental drug.

Question: What ethical steps should be taken before granting access to an experimental treatment?

Answer: Confirm potential benefit, ensure informed consent, and follow regulatory and institutional protocols.

Explanation: Compassionate use must balance patient autonomy, safety, and evidence. Clear communication about risks, uncertainties, and alternatives is essential before proceeding.

Elderly Abuse in Long-Term Care

Scenario: A nurse in a long-term care facility notices bruises on an elderly resident's arms and overhears a personal support worker speaking harshly to them. The patient is reluctant to talk about it.

Question: What should the nurse do?

Answer: Report the suspected abuse to the facility administration and the appropriate provincial reporting body immediately.

Explanation: Healthcare providers are legally and ethically obligated to report suspected elder abuse to protect vulnerable patients. This ensures safety and initiates an investigation.

Genetic Testing and Privacy

Scenario: A patient undergoes genetic testing and the results indicate a high risk for a hereditary cancer. The patient requests that this information not be shared with family members, despite potential implications for their health.

Question: What should the physician prioritize in handling this situation?

Answer: Respect patient confidentiality while discussing the benefits of disclosure.

Explanation: Genetic information is sensitive and protected by privacy laws. Physicians should maintain confidentiality but also educate the patient on the potential health benefits of informing family members.

Global Health Ethics – Providing Care in Low-Resource Settings

Scenario: A Canadian physician volunteers in a rural African clinic where resources are scarce. They must decide how to allocate the limited supply of antibiotics among many sick children.

Question: What ethical principle should guide the physician's decision?

Answer: Justice – fair distribution of limited resources.

Explanation: In low-resource settings, physicians must prioritize patients based on medical need, urgency, and potential benefit, while ensuring fairness and equity in resource allocation.

Informed Consent

Scenario: A 45-year-old patient is scheduled for elective knee replacement. The surgeon explains the procedure but omits discussing a rare but serious complication—nerve damage.

Question: Is the consent valid if a significant risk was not disclosed?

Answer: No.

Explanation: For consent to be valid, patients must be informed of all significant risks, benefits, and alternatives. Omitting a material risk undermines informed decision-making.

Informed Consent in Pediatric Care – Parental vs. Child Decision Rights

Scenario: A 15-year-old refuses a recommended treatment, but their parents insist on proceeding.

Question: Who has the final decision in this situation?

Answer: It depends on the child's maturity and legal capacity; a mature minor may have the right to refuse treatment.

Explanation: Ethically and legally, competent minors may have decision-making authority if they demonstrate sufficient understanding. Physicians must assess capacity and involve ethics/legal consultation if needed.

Mandatory Reporting (e.g., Child Abuse, Elder Abuse)

Scenario: A physician suspects that a child's repeated injuries are the result of physical abuse.

Question: What is the physician's legal obligation?

Answer: Report the suspicion to the appropriate child protection authority immediately.

Explanation: Mandatory reporting laws require healthcare providers to report suspected abuse, regardless of confirmation, to protect vulnerable individuals from harm.

Managing Medical Errors and Disclosure

Scenario: A family physician realizes that they prescribed the wrong dosage of a medication to a patient, which could cause significant side effects. The patient has not yet started the medication.

Question: What should the physician do after identifying the error?

Answer: Immediately inform the patient about the error, explain potential risks, correct the prescription, and document the disclosure.

Explanation: Ethical medical practice requires transparency when errors occur. Prompt disclosure helps maintain trust, prevents harm, and aligns with professional standards of honesty.

Medical Assistance in Dying (MAiD)

Scenario: A 72-year-old man with end-stage COPD meets all legal eligibility criteria for MAiD in his jurisdiction. He requests it to avoid prolonged suffering.

Question: What is the physician's primary ethical responsibility in this scenario?

Answer: Ensure all eligibility criteria are met and the decision is voluntary.

Explanation: The physician must verify capacity, voluntariness, informed consent, and adherence to legal safeguards before proceeding with MAiD.

Patient Refusal of Treatment

Scenario: A competent adult patient with pneumonia refuses antibiotic treatment despite understanding the risks, including death.

Question: Can the physician proceed with treatment without consent?

Answer: No, the physician must respect the patient's decision.

Explanation: Competent patients have the right to refuse treatment, even if the decision may result in serious harm or death. Physicians should document the discussion and ensure informed refusal.

Physician-Assisted Suicide vs. Euthanasia Distinctions

Scenario: A terminally ill patient asks their physician about ending their life under medical supervision.

Question: What is the key ethical distinction between physician-assisted suicide and euthanasia?

Answer: In physician-assisted suicide, the patient self-administers the lethal medication; in euthanasia, the physician directly administers it.

Explanation: Understanding the distinction is important because legal and ethical frameworks vary, with different safeguards, documentation, and consent requirements.

Physician Conscientious Objection

Scenario: A family physician refuses to prescribe contraception due to personal religious beliefs.

Question: What is the ethical obligation toward the patient?

Answer: Provide an effective referral to another provider who can offer the requested service without causing undue delay.

Explanation: Conscientious objection is permitted, but physicians must not abandon the patient. Referral ensures patient access to legally available medical care.

Privacy Breaches and Data Security

Scenario: A nurse accidentally sends a patient's lab results to the wrong email address due to a typographical error.

Question: What is the immediate ethical and professional obligation in this situation?

Answer: Notify the patient and the privacy officer immediately, investigate the breach, and take corrective measures to prevent recurrence.

Explanation: Healthcare providers have a duty to protect patient confidentiality. When breaches occur, rapid notification, transparency, and system improvements are essential to minimize harm and prevent future incidents.

Professional Boundaries

Scenario: A physician begins receiving frequent personal text messages from a patient that are unrelated to medical care.

Question: What is the appropriate action for the physician?

Answer: Set clear limits and redirect communication to professional channels.

Explanation: Maintaining professional boundaries protects the integrity of the physician–patient relationship and prevents potential ethical or legal issues.

Research Ethics and Human Subjects Protection

Scenario: A clinical trial seeks volunteers for a new cancer therapy, but the risks are not fully explained to participants.

Question: What is the ethical obligation of the researcher?

Answer: Ensure that informed consent is obtained by fully disclosing all known risks, benefits, and alternatives before participation.

Explanation: Ethical research requires voluntary participation based on comprehensive understanding of potential risks and benefits. Transparency protects participants and upholds research integrity.

Reporting Impaired or Incompetent Colleagues

Scenario: A nurse notices that a physician frequently appears drowsy during shifts and makes several prescribing errors.

Question: What is the physician's ethical obligation in this scenario?

Answer: To report the concern to the appropriate regulatory or supervisory body while maintaining patient safety and confidentiality.

Explanation: Healthcare providers have an ethical duty to protect patients from harm, which includes reporting colleagues whose impairment or incompetence may compromise care. Reporting should follow institutional policy and protect both patients and due process for the colleague.

Sexual Harassment and Discrimination

Scenario: A junior physician reports to you that a senior colleague made repeated inappropriate comments about their appearance during clinical rounds.

Question: What is the appropriate immediate action?

Answer: Address the safety of the junior physician, document the report, and escalate the matter to human resources or the appropriate regulatory body.

Explanation: Sexual harassment violates professional conduct standards and workplace safety. Prompt reporting and intervention protect the complainant and uphold a respectful work environment.

Social Media Use by Physicians – Boundaries and Professional Image

Scenario: A physician posts a case on social media without patient identifiers, but colleagues feel the details could still allow patient recognition.

Question: What should the physician do before posting clinical cases on social media?

Answer: Ensure full de-identification, obtain patient consent if possible, and follow professional guidelines for online conduct.

Explanation: Even without names, clinical details can sometimes identify patients. Maintaining confidentiality and professional integrity is essential to preserve trust and comply with privacy laws.

Surrogate Decision-Making

Scenario: An unconscious patient has no advance directive. Their spouse insists on pursuing aggressive treatment, while their adult child believes the patient would have wanted comfort-focused care.

Question: Who should make the medical decisions?

Answer: The legally designated substitute decision-maker, typically the spouse.

Explanation: In most jurisdictions, the spouse has legal priority as the surrogate decision-maker unless otherwise specified. The physician should guide decisions based on the patient's known or inferred wishes.

Telemedicine and Digital Health Ethics

Scenario: A rural patient consults a specialist via telemedicine, but the internet connection is unstable, affecting communication.

Question: What is the physician's ethical obligation in this scenario?

Answer: Ensure informed consent about limitations and arrange alternative care if necessary.

Explanation: Ethically, physicians must disclose telemedicine's limitations, protect patient confidentiality, and ensure quality of care comparable to in-person visits.

Truth-Telling vs. Therapeutic Privilege

Scenario: A patient with severe depression is diagnosed with a terminal illness. The physician worries that telling the truth will worsen their mental state.

Question: Is it ethical to withhold the diagnosis under therapeutic privilege?

Answer: Only in rare cases and for a short duration.

Explanation: Therapeutic privilege allows temporary withholding of information to prevent serious harm, but full disclosure should occur as soon as it is safe and appropriate.

Use of Restraints (Physical and Chemical)

Scenario: An agitated patient in the emergency department is at risk of harming themselves and others. The team considers applying soft wrist restraints and administering a sedative.

Question: What is the ethical priority before using restraints?

Answer: Use the least restrictive measure necessary, ensuring patient safety and dignity.

Explanation: Ethically, restraints should be a last resort, applied only when less restrictive interventions have failed and there is immediate risk of harm. Ongoing monitoring is essential.

Healthcare providers have a duty to protect patient confidentiality. When breaches occur, rapid notification, transparency, and system improvements are essential to minimize harm and prevent future incidents.

Whistleblowing – Ethical and Legal Protections for Healthcare Providers

Scenario: A respiratory therapist discovers that a colleague is falsifying patient ventilator records to hide treatment errors.

Question: What is the ethically correct course of action?

Answer: Report the misconduct through the appropriate internal or external channels.

Explanation: Whistleblowing is justified when patient safety is at risk. Many jurisdictions provide legal protection to healthcare workers who report unsafe or unethical practices in good faith.

Whistleblowing – Ethical and Legal Protections for Healthcare Providers

Scenario: A respiratory therapist discovers that a colleague is falsifying patient ventilator records to hide treatment errors.

Question: What is the ethically correct course of action?

Answer: Report the misconduct through the appropriate internal or external channels.

Explanation: Whistleblowing is justified when patient safety is at risk. Many jurisdictions provide legal protection to healthcare workers who report unsafe or unethical practices in good faith.

Workplace Bullying and Professional Respect in Healthcare Teams

Scenario: A nurse reports that a senior physician frequently belittles junior staff during rounds, creating a hostile work environment.

Question: What is the most appropriate first step?

Answer: Report the behavior to hospital administration or HR for investigation.

Explanation: Workplace bullying violates professional respect and can harm team performance and patient care. Reporting ensures accountability and promotes a safe workplace.

www.ingramcontent.com/pod-product-compliance
Lightning Source LLC
Chambersburg PA
CBHW040928210326
41597CB00030B/5218